A Call to Action

Advancing Essential Services and Research on Fetal Alcohol Spectrum Disorders

A Report of the National Task Force on
Fetal Alcohol Syndrome and Fetal Alcohol Effect

Prepared by:
National Task Force on Fetal Alcohol Syndrome and
Fetal Alcohol Effect Post Exposure Writing Group
Heather Carmichael Olson, PhD
Melinda M. Ohlemiller, BA, MA
Mary J. O'Connor, PhD, ABPP
Carole W. Brown, EdD
Colleen A. Morris, MD
Karla Damus, RN, PhD

March 2009

CONTENTS

ACKNOWLEDGEMENTS

Special thanks go to the following individuals for the development of this report.

National Task Force on Fetal Alcohol Syndrome and Fetal Alcohol Effect - Members: Jean A. Wright, MD (Chair), Backus Children's Hospital, Savannah, GA; Kristen L. Barry, PhD, Department of Veterans Affairs and University of Michigan, Ann Arbor, Michigan; James E. Berner, MD, Alaska Native Tribal Health Consortium; Carole W. Brown, EdD, Catholic University of America; Raul Caetano, MD, PhD, MPH, University of Texas School of Public Health; Grace Chang, MD, MPH, Brigham and Women's Hospital, Boston, MA; Mary C. DeJoseph, DO, Philadelphia College of Osteopathic Medicine; Lisa A. Miller, MD, MSPH, Colorado Department of Public Health and Environment; Colleen A. Morris, MD, University of Nevada School of Medicine; Mary J. O'Connor, PhD, University of California at Los Angeles School of Medicine; Melinda M. Ohlemiller, BA, MA, Nurses for Newborns Foundation (formerly of the Saint Louis Arc); Heather Carmichael Olson, PhD, University of Washington, School of Medicine; Kenneth R. Warren, PhD, National Institute on Alcohol Abuse and Alcoholism (NIAAA), National Institutes of Health (NIH)

Liaison Representatives: George Brenneman, MD, FAAP, American Academy of Pediatrics; Karla Damus, RN, PhD, March of Dimes; George A. Hacker, JD, Center for Science in the Public Interest; Kathleen T. Mitchell, MHS, LCADC, National Organization on Fetal Alcohol Syndrome; Sharon Davis, PhD, Arc of the United States; Robert J. Sokol, MD, American College of Obstetricians and Gynecologists

Post-Exposure Working Group Members (Past and Present): George Brenneman, MD, FAAP, American Academy of Pediatrics; Carole W. Brown, EdD, Catholic University of America; Faye Calhoun, PhD, Former Deputy Director, NIAAA and consultant to NIAAA; Deborah E. Cohen, PhD (co-chair), New Jersey Department of Human Services, Trenton, NJ; Sharon Davis, PhD, Arc of the United States; Callie Gass, FASD Center for Excellence, Substance Abuse and Mental Health Services Administration (SAMHSA); Colleen A. Morris, MD, University of Nevada School of Medicine; Mary J. O'Connor, PhD (co-chair), University of California at Los Angeles School of Medicine; Melinda M. Ohlemiller, Saint Louis Arc; Heather Carmichael Olson, PhD (co-chair), University of Washington, School of Medicine; Charles M. Schad, EdD, Retired Educator, Spearfish, South Dakota; Jacquelyn Bertrand, PhD, National Center on Birth Defects and Developmental Disabilities (NCBDDD), Centers for Disease Control and Prevention (CDC); Elizabeth Parra Dang, MPH, NCBDDD, CDC Post-Exposure Writing Group: Heather Carmichael Olson, PhD, University of Washington, School of Medicine; Melinda M. Ohlemiller, BA, MA, Nurses for Newborns Foundation (formerly of the Saint Louis Arc); Mary J. O'Connor, PhD, University of California at Los Angeles School of Medicine; Carole W. Brown, EdD, Catholic University of America; Colleen A. Morris, MD, University of Nevada School of Medicine; Karla Damus, RN, PhD, March of Dimes

Additional Reviewers and Consultants: Jacquelyn Bertrand, PhD, NCBDDD, CDC; R. Louise Floyd, DSN, RN, NCBDDD, CDC; Mary Kate Weber, MPH, NCBDDD, CDC; Coleen Boyle, PhD, NCBDDD, CDC; José F. Cordero, MD, MPH, University of Puerto Rico School of Public Health (formerly Director of NCBDDD, CDC); Kathleen T. Mitchell, MHS, LCADC, National Organization on Fetal Alcohol Syndrome; Robert J. Sokol, MD, American College of Obstetricians and Gynecologists; Kenneth R. Warren, PhD, NIAAA, NIH

Appreciation to: the Winokur and Welch families for sharing their photos
(Cover: Donnie, Iyal and Morasha Winokur; Page 3: Debbie and Erin Welch).

INTRODUCTION

In 2004, the National Task Force on Fetal Alcohol Syndrome and Fetal Alcohol Effect, coordinated by the Centers for Disease Control and Prevention's National Center on Birth Defects and Developmental Disabilities, established a working group committed to addressing the needs of individuals living with fetal alcohol spectrum disorders (FASDs) and their families. The culmination of this working group's discussions and Task Force deliberations is reflected in this Call to Action report. The document highlights ten recommendations to improve and expand efforts regarding early identification, diagnostic services, and quality research on interventions for individuals with FASDs and their families. Additional background information is provided to support these recommendations and to further educate readers on the topic of FASDs, progress to date, and what still needs to be done to support individuals with FASDs. The intent of this report is to guide federal, state and local agencies, researchers and clinicians, family support groups, and other partners on actions needed to advance essential services for individuals with FASDs and their families and to promote continued intervention research efforts.

A CALL TO ACTION

Fetal alcohol spectrum disorders (FASDs) are serious, lifelong birth defects and developmental disabilities caused by prenatal alcohol exposure. They are 100% preventable. Still, a surprisingly large number of children are born with FASDs each year.

FASDs are a public health problem we must face. The U.S. Surgeon General has stated clearly that no amount of alcohol consumption can be considered safe for a pregnant woman and that alcohol can damage a fetus at any stage of pregnancy (Office of the Surgeon General, 2005). Yet, recent U.S. surveys reveal that approximately 12% of pregnant women still drink alcohol (CDC, 2004; SAMHSA, 2007). This means 1 in 8 fetuses are exposed to alcohol and placed at risk for FASDs. Maternal alcohol use is a growing worldwide phenomenon. It affects children and families of all ethnicities in all societies. Important international collaborative research is beginning to describe the alarming scope of this problem. While community and professional awareness of FASDs have increased, expanded awareness and informed action are sorely needed.

FASDs cause a range of lasting medical and developmental problems and result in economic losses of billions of dollars.

FASDs can also mean long-standing suffering for families. FASDs are considered both medical conditions and developmental disabilities. They include a wide range of conditions, from subtle neurodevelopmental impairments to the full fetal alcohol syndrome (FAS). Individuals with FASDs can have physical, mental, behavioral, and/or learning disabilities with possible lifelong implications. Research shows that individuals with FASDs often have significant, long-term deficits in functional life skills. These deficits lead to problems with day-to-day functioning as well as health care issues, including birth defects and increased risk for injury, unintended pregnancy, and sexually transmitted diseases. FASDs can also be associated with mental health difficulties, disrupted school and job experiences, trouble with the law, difficulties with independent living, substance abuse, problems with parenting, and more (Bertrand et al., 2004; Streissguth et al., 2004). The median adjusted annual cost of fetal alcohol syndrome has been estimated at $3.6 billion, but the costs associated with the entire fetal alcohol spectrum are surely much higher.

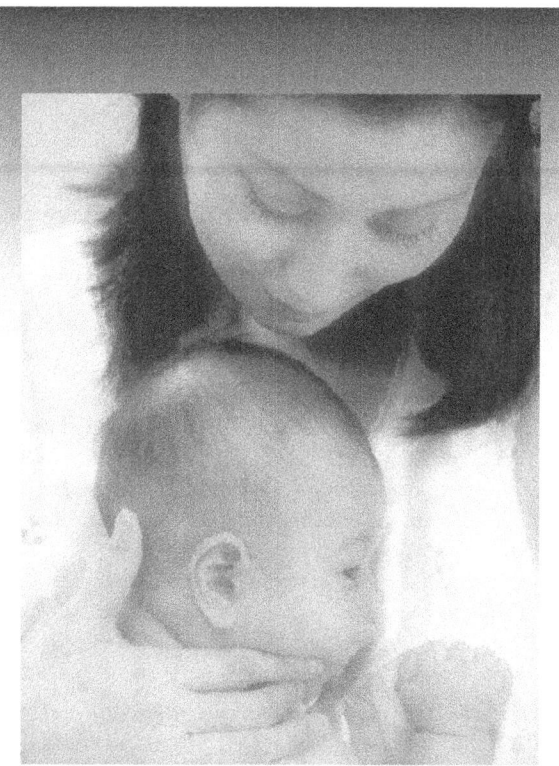

Early, appropriate diagnosis of FASDs is a vital first step to improving outcomes for affected individuals and their families.

There is an emerging consensus on how to define FASDs; however, much research is needed to reach a diagnostic standard and to delineate the entire fetal alcohol spectrum. Diagnostic capacity is growing yet still insufficient in the United States, Canada, and abroad. For this reason, many individuals with FASDs are unrecognized or misdiagnosed. Efforts are ongoing to create and use standardized, reliable diagnostic systems across the globe and to continually improve guidelines as new knowledge emerges from research.

Expert opinion from treating professionals, a wealth of family experience, compelling animal research, and pioneering intervention studies indicate that appropriate treatment of FASDs can have a measurable, positive impact.

At the present time, even when appropriately diagnosed, individuals with FASDs often receive treatment that is incomplete or inappropriate. Without suitable treatment and interventions, individuals with FASDs may never reach their full potential. Not providing suitable treatment can also result in unnecessary costs as individuals enter systems (such as juvenile justice) with problems that data suggest could have been averted by earlier intervention. Families of affected individuals also need support within the medical and health care systems, and in early intervention and education, juvenile justice and corrections, substance abuse treatment, mental health systems, and social services.

Fortunately, it is possible to define and address the treatment problems raised by FASDs. Because of increasing societal concern, especially over the past 10 years, important steps have been taken and the need for further action made very clear. In the United States, needs assessments have taken place through nationwide public town hall meetings and community agency initiatives (Ryan, Bonnett & Gass, 2006). Intervention guidelines for FASDs are evolving in the United States, Canada, England, and other countries around the world. Strategic research plans are in place to stimulate better description of the entire fetal alcohol spectrum, hone diagnosis, and explain mechanisms of alcohol's action on the developing child's body and brain so that biomarkers and targeted treatments can be identified. An important but limited program of systematic FASD intervention research has begun in the United States and abroad.

Collaboration between government agencies, professional organizations, researchers, and families is needed to adequately address FASDs.

In 2000, the United States Congress initiated a national forum for discussion of FASDs and interagency coordination at the federal level. Building on existing research, and advised by experts and parents, federal leaders have put in place strategic research plans for funding the study of FASDs. To promote further organized action, the Substance Abuse and Mental Health Services Administration's (SAMHSA) FASD Center for Excellence has compiled a comprehensive database of available educational materials and products, research on FASDs, field-initiated efforts to educate professionals and the public, and community-based and/or research-driven efforts to provide services. Appendices B through F provide information on the efforts of the National Task Force on Fetal Alcohol Syndrome and Fetal Alcohol Effect, National Institute on Alcohol Abuse and Alcoholism (NIAAA), Centers for Disease Control and Prevention (CDC), SAMHSA through their FASD Center for Excellence, and the Interagency Coordinating Committee on FAS (ICCFAS).

The groundwork has been laid to confront the serious public health problem presented by FASDs. It is reasonable, efficient, and humane to establish an integrated system of services for individuals and families affected by these conditions. This is a problem that can be dealt with, but momentum must be sustained. What is needed is well-informed public policy on FASDs and a clear, ongoing societal commitment to advancing research and ensuring essential services for persons with FASDs and their caregivers.

RECOMMENDATIONS

The National Task Force on Fetal Alcohol Syndrome and Fetal Alcohol Effect has developed the following recommendations to respond to the need for essential services for and research on FASDs. Specific action steps to carry out these recommendations are found in Appendix A.

1. Modify eligibility and diagnostic classification systems to include FASDs so as to recognize FASDs as approved conditions under all federal disability-related benefit programs.
2. Improve diagnostic access by setting up screening systems for FASDs and increasing professional multidisciplinary diagnostic capacity in communities.
3. Intensify research initiatives and interagency coordination to:
   - delineate the full fetal alcohol spectrum,
   - continue study of alcohol mechanisms and biomarkers,
   - carry out longitudinal descriptive studies,
   - establish effective interventions,
   - translate interventions to the community, and
   - improve the quality and utilization of interventions in all service systems for those with FASDs.
4. Promote a comprehensive and accessible continuum of care for families raising infants, children, and adolescents with FASDs.
5. Promote a comprehensive and accessible continuum of care for youth, adults, and older individuals with FASDs.
6. Encourage comprehensive professional education on FASDs, and assessment of knowledge gained, within multiple service systems.
7. Enhance strong, collaborative, interagency leadership at state and national levels (that includes parent representation) to inform legislators, policymakers, and the public.
8. Recognize grassroots family support and advocacy organizations focused on FASDs, which are powerful and efficient agents of change.
9. Improve ongoing national surveillance systems to identify individuals with FASDs to better track prevalence, provide needed intervention, and assess the impact of prevention programs.
10. Maintain a national forum in which parents, advocates, professional organizations, and experts in the field of FASDs can work to advance essential services and research for individuals with FASDs and their families.

FASDs

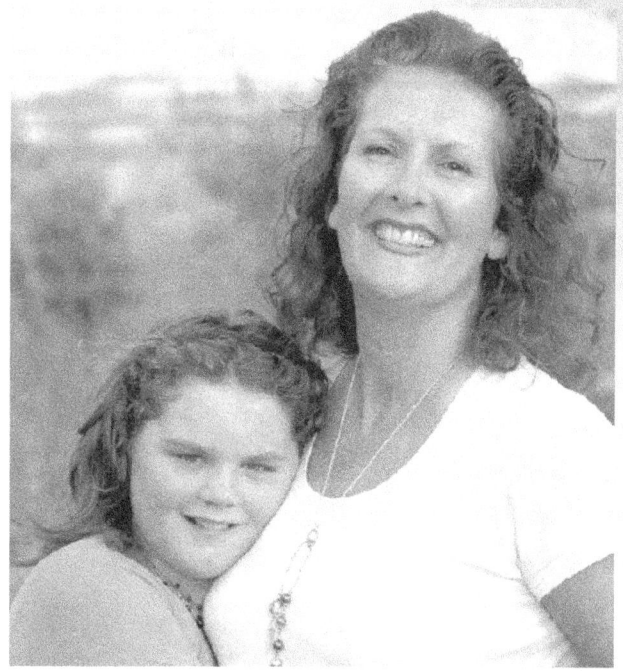

FREQUENTLY ASKED QUESTIONS

What are FASDs?

FASDs are increasingly understood as a spectrum or continuum of effects found across many aspects of physical development, learning, and function (Warren et al., 2004). Individuals with FASDs can, but do not always, show adverse physical signs, such as characteristic facial anomalies or other body malformations. The learning and functional effects of prenatal alcohol exposure are the most troubling and difficult (but important) to identify, diagnose, and treat. These effects vary not only in type, but in severity. Some individuals can be mildly affected in one area of learning or behavior, but moderately or severely affected in another area. The range of FASDs includes the full fetal alcohol syndrome (FAS). Although FAS is found in a fairly small proportion of children affected by prenatal alcohol exposure, it is most easily diagnosed. Unfortunately, the effects of alcohol are not readily recognized if they do not fit the classic FAS definition. A larger number of children, adolescents, and adults have prenatal alcohol–induced impairments that can be just as serious, or more so, than those seen in people with FAS (Kodituwakku, 2007; Mattson, Riley, Gramling, Delis & Jones, 1998; Riley & McGee, 2005). The terms "partial FAS" and "alcohol-related neurodevelopmental disorder" (ARND) have been applied to these conditions, along with other diagnostic terms. In addition, some children prenatally-exposed to alcohol are born without the characteristic facial features of FAS, but have other alcohol-related physical abnormalities of the skeleton and certain organ systems. These anomalies are referred to as "alcohol-related birth defects" (ARBD) (Alcohol Research & Health, 2000; Stratton, Howe & Battaglia, 1996).

How does alcohol affect fetal development?

Alcohol is a neurobehavioral teratogen—a substance that through prenatal exposure affects the body and (most importantly) the brain of a developing fetus. Alcohol alters how neurons and connections between neurons are formed. It also affects development at the cellular, hormonal, neurochemical, structural, and functional levels. It is thought that alcohol exposure affects fetal programming, laying the groundwork for atypical development and adverse life outcomes. Extensive animal research, long-term human descriptive studies, clinical studies, and neuroimaging research all come together to clearly show the lifelong negative impact that alcohol use during pregnancy can have on the developing child (Burden, Jacobson & Jacobson, 2005; Gemma, Vichi & Testai, 2007; Hannigan, O'Leary-Moore, & Berman, 2007; Kodituwakku, 2007; Miller & Spear, 2006; Sokol et al., 2007; Spadoni, McKee, Fryer & Riley, 2007; Streissguth et al., 2004; Zhang, Sliwowska & Weinberg, 2005).

How common are FASDs?

In the United States, FASDs are now known to have a higher prevalence rate than previously thought and to occur across all ethnicities. The reported rates of FAS vary widely, depending on the population studied and surveillance methods used. CDC studies show FAS rates ranging from 0.2 to 1.5 cases per 1,000 live births. Such rates are comparable with or above other common developmental disabilities such as Down Syndrome or Spina Bifida (Bertrand et al., 2004). Other alcohol-related conditions resulting from prenatal exposure, such as partial FAS, ARND, and ARBD, are believed to occur about three times as often as FAS (Sampson et al., 1997). But the full extent of the problem is still under investigation, and improved prevalence studies are needed. Some have estimated the rates of the full range of FASDs as high as 9 or 10 per 1,000 live births (May & Gossage, 2001; Sampson et al., 1997). Reasonable estimates translate to about 40,000 alcohol-impacted births in the United States each year (Lupton, Burd & Harwood, 2004). FASDs are also a global health problem. FASDs are found worldwide, usually at rates similar to those in the United States. But some countries with even higher prevalence rates have reached out for guidance and collaboration in research efforts to address FASDs. Many nations have had long-standing concern about FASDs, and there is now emerging alarm in countries that had not previously recognized the problem. (Viljoen et al., 2005; May et al., 2006).

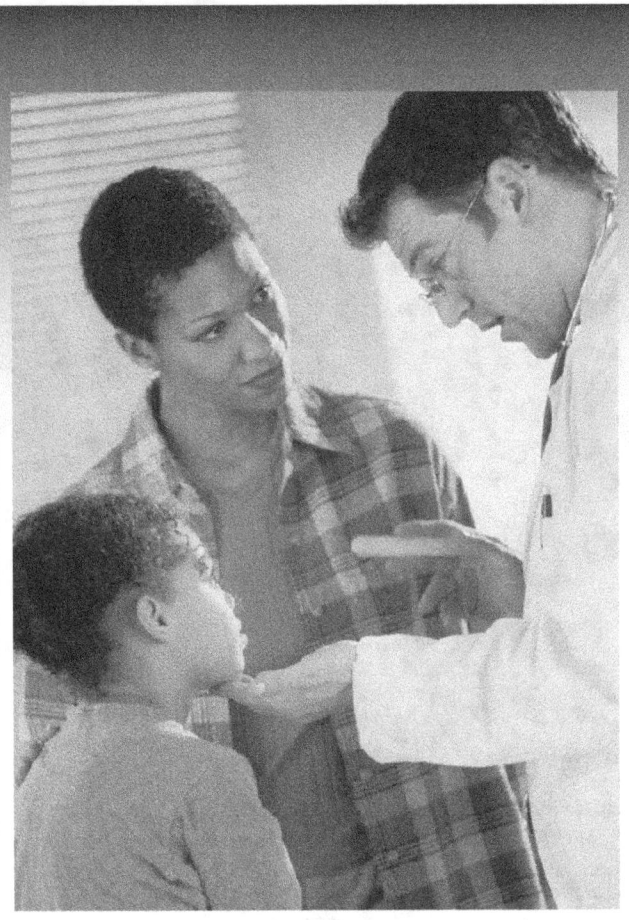

What are the costs of FASDs? The costs of FASDs are both human and financial. The human costs of FASDs arise from the debilitating secondary disabilities found among affected individuals, and the emotional and financial burdens on their families—made clear in nationwide town hall meetings that took place from 2002 to 2005 (Ryan, Bonnett & Gass, 2006). For instance, parents raising children with clearly diagnosed FASDs report clinically elevated levels of stress (Paley, O'Connor, Frankel & Marquardt, 2006). Careful estimates of economic cost data in the United States for the full fetal alcohol syndrome (FAS) reveal that it is one of the most costly birth defects. Lupton and colleagues (2004) estimated that the median adjusted annual cost of FAS to the U.S. economy is $3.6 billion. They also estimated that the adjusted total lifetime cost per individual with FAS (as of 2002 and updated based on the medical services price index) was $2.9 million. Annual state cost estimates vary depending on population and female at-risk drinking rates. More details on published cost studies can be found on SAMHSA's FASD Center for Excellence website (www.fasdcenter.samhsa.gov). Little is known about costs of the wider fetal alcohol spectrum beyond FAS, but additional affected individuals can only further raise societal costs and caregiving burden.

Where Are We Now in Responding to FASDs? Prevention of FASDs and community education remain important.

Pregnant women are advised to abstain from all alcohol use, a long-standing federal advisory that is also supported by major professional societies (e.g., American College of Obstetricians & Gynecologists, 2005). However, studies conducted by the CDC (2004) and SAMHSA (2007) found that 12% of pregnant women reported consuming alcohol, with 2-3% reporting binge drinking (5 or more drinks per drinking occasion). Of the approximately 4 million live births in the United States per year, this translates to almost a half million women consuming alcohol during pregnancy with an estimated 80,000-120,000 women drinking alcohol at levels that place their babies at increased risk for adverse outcomes. In another study, approximately 3% of pregnant women reported drinking at levels that have been consistently associated with adverse effects on the fetus (Jacobson & Jacobson, 1999). Also, more than half of all women of childbearing age (18 through 44 years of age) reported alcohol use, and approximately one in eight reported binge drinking in the past month (CDC, 2004; SAMHSA, 2007). Given that half of U.S. pregnancies are unplanned (Finer & Henshaw, 2006), this rate of drinking among women of childbearing age poses a substantial risk for FASDs.

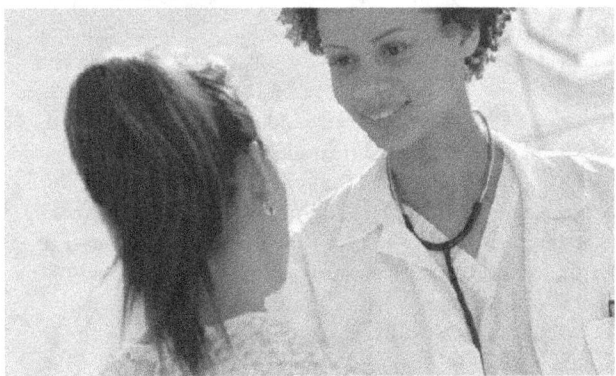

In response to this public health concern, a clinical plan of action for reducing adverse outcomes from prenatal alcohol exposure has been proposed (Floyd, O'Connor, Bertrand & Sokol, 2006). Some progress has been made in preventing FASDs, although prevention must remain a major aim. Educational approaches on screening for and preventing women's drinking have been developed. Both brief and indicated, longer-term preventive treatment methods have been tested. The National Task Force on Fetal Alcohol Syndrome and Fetal Alcohol Affect recently reviewed the evidence to date on effective prevention methods to reduce alcohol use and alcohol-exposed pregnancies— and developed recommendations to inform future research, practice, and public policy regarding prevention of FASDs (Barry et al.,

2009). Community awareness of FASDs has increased, but must expand. A broad range of educational materials have been created, and these materials need wider dissemination. Importantly, pivotal federal task forces and professional societies are beginning to take a stand on prevention of FASDs and producing guidelines for how to respond (e.g., American Academy of Pediatrics, 2000; American College of Obstetricians & Gynecologists, 2006; NIAAA, 2005; U.S. Preventive Services Task Force, 2004).

Prevention of FASDs can be achieved. Evidence is accumulating that preventive intervention can reduce prenatal alcohol use and increase family planning efforts (e.g., Chang, McNamara & Orav, 2005; Floyd et al., 2007; Grant, Ernst, Streissguth & Stark, 2005; O'Connor & Whaley, 2007). It is important to assess different preventive approaches (universal, selective, and indicated) targeting different types of populations (Hankin, 2002), and to study the success of multi-level, community-wide prevention efforts. Continuing, definitive prevention research, including innovations such as the study of neuroprotective agents, is crucial. But prevention of FASDs cannot be the only response to this set of developmental disabilities.

Accurate detection and expanded diagnosis of FASDs are essential. Even with prevention efforts, many children are born with FASDs and need diagnosis and appropriate intervention across the lifespan. Their families, schools, service systems, and larger communities need support and effective, practical ways to respond. Surveillance programs and research are underway to understand women's drinking and rates of FAS. There are small but lively research programs studying biomarkers and alcohol exposure ascertainment. This research will allow better screening and detection in pregnancy or early infancy. Researchers are actively studying the reliability of existing FASD diagnostic systems, while also collaborating to improve diagnostic methodology through technology such as imaging and both 2-D and 3-D facial modeling. Research to case-define disorders along the entire fetal alcohol spectrum is underway, using behavioral and physical methodologies, including brain imaging. Better case definitions will allow more precise estimates of prevalence across the full range of FASDs. In particular, there is a crucial need to case-define alcohol-related neurodevelopmental disorder (ARND), which has not yet been adequately described, although research is actively being pursued. These promising research programs must continue in order to expand and build momentum to accomplish the goals of precision in estimating prevalence and incidence; in detecting prenatal alcohol exposure and the possible presence of FASDs as early as possible; and in developing clear diagnoses. Meanwhile, though, useful diagnostic guidelines do exist (e.g., Bertrand et al., 2004; Chudley et al., 2005). Practical and increasingly widely used diagnostic systems that can describe the full range of alcohol-related disabilities are in use, and successful models for diagnostic clinics do exist. What is urgently needed is a significant increase in FASD diagnostic capacity and accessibility.

Intervention for individuals with FASDs is a high priority. There is real hope that with appropriate and early intervention, children with FASDs can have improved outcomes. Basic animal research and human studies are building the case that diagnosis and intervention can change outcome. Research on animal models of FAS suggests that there is neuronal plasticity and that appropriate environmental enrichment and motor training has potential to improve behavioral and learning outcomes and reduce alcohol-induced injury to the brain and central nervous system. This is thought to be especially true early in life, but even to occur during the animal equivalent of adolescence or early adulthood (e.g., Hannigan et al., 2007). Animal research suggests that pharmacological treatments may also have positive effects (e.g., Vaglenova et al., 2007). Natural history research on clinical human samples highlights "protective factors" that are related to reduced odds that negative outcomes in functional life skills will occur among individuals with FASDs (Streissguth et al., 2004). These protective factors can be enhanced through intervention.

Infant mental health studies and early intervention research among children with a variety of developmental disabilities suggest strong potential for positive change if intervention is designed on the basis of current scientific data about child development and early psychopathology (Olson, Jirikowic, Kartin & Astley, 2007). Treatment in the school years or adolescence can likely improve educational outcomes and functional life skills, and prevent or reduce secondary disabilities and debilitating family strife (Coles, Strickland, Padgett & Bellmoff, 2006; Kalberg & Buckley, 2007). Indeed, recent carefully controlled FASD intervention studies in the United States show positive effects for school-age children and families (Coles et al., 2009; Interventions for Children with FASDs Research Consortium, in press; Kable et al., 2007; O'Connor et al., 2006; Olson et al., 2005), and pilot studies in the United States and abroad show promise (e.g., Adnams et al., 2007). Even as late as adulthood, diagnosis and intervention for individuals with FASDs are deemed crucial (especially holistic treatment and management of associated mental disorders), and can likely reduce suffering and cost to affected individuals and those who care for them (Streissguth & O'Malley, 2000). Many promising intervention ideas exist, and parents and providers are discussing what is needed within the full continuum of services (Olson, 2006). Some field-initiated intervention projects are also underway in the United States (see SAMHSA's FASD Center for Excellence [www.fasdcenter.samhsa.gov] and CDC websites [www.cdc.gov/ncbddd/fas]), and several international cooperative projects for prevention and intervention with FASDs are operating, as part of global outreach to resource-poor countries (Calhoun et al., 2006). But these services and beginning intervention research are truly only a foundation. Much work remains to be done in the high-priority, under-funded, and relatively unexplored area of intervention for FASDs. Intervention research should become a major focus in the field of FASDs. Research should be programmatic and, when possible, conducted in randomized control trials, and held to standards that will generate an appropriate evidence base.

Ongoing communication and cooperation between government, professional organizations, researchers, and families are imperative.

The basic systems needed to ensure advancement in the field of FASDs do exist, and it is imperative that these systems be maintained. Since the mid 1970s, student and senior basic scientists, animal researchers, and clinical investigators interested in FASDs have met together as the FASD Study Group (see http://rsoa.org/fas.html). This research interchange, which began spontaneously, now includes efficient interaction with agencies interested in FASDs, has been encouraged by the NIAAA, and has resulted in faster research progress. There is currently a productive and wide-ranging research environment exploring FASDs, although the number of researchers remains relatively small (Bonthius, Olson & Thomas, 2006). The NIAAA and CDC have agendas for research on FASDs (see Appendices C and D). Family advocacy groups have increasingly coalesced across the United States and abroad, including the National Organization on Fetal Alcohol Syndrome (NOFAS), which recently gathered an FASD Congressional Caucus (see www.nofas.org). In the last 10 years, increasing cooperation on many other levels has boosted progress on the public health problem of FASDs. In 2000, Congress mandated creation of the National Task Force on Fetal Alcohol Syndrome and Fetal Alcohol Effect with participation from governmental agencies and research funding bodies, professional organizations, family advocacy groups, and experts in the field of FASDs, with Task Force activities open to public comment (sunset for the Task Force occurred in 2007; see Appendix B). In 2001, SAMHSA's FASD Center for Excellence was created with multiple initiatives, and with impetus from the public, has fortunately been refunded by SAMHSA (see Appendix E). In 1996, the Interagency Coordinating Committee on FAS (ICCFAS) was created,

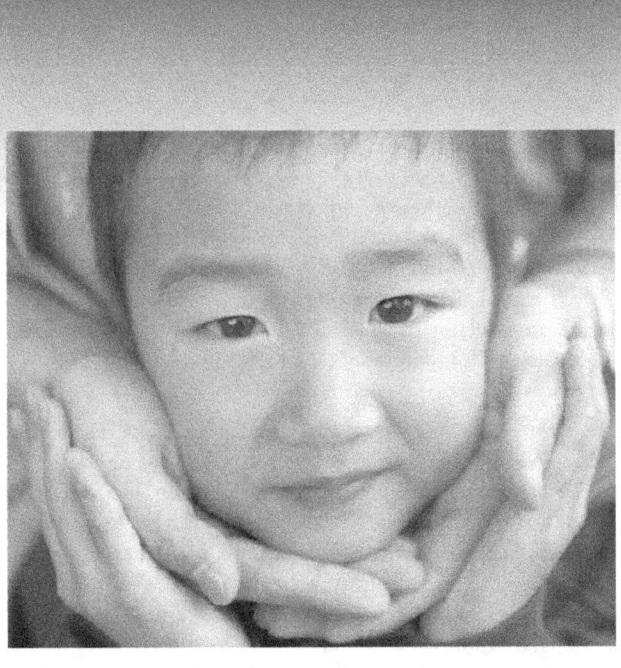

with participation by decision-makers in the many service systems affected by FASDs (see Appendix F). Experience has shown that communication and cooperation in this field can function well, inspire creativity, enhance efficiency, and drive progress. Collaboration and integration in research, practice, and public policy must continue.

What are the Next Steps?

Now is the time to build on earlier momentum and renew efforts to meet the challenge of FASDs. This is a call to action. Without continued momentum, public will could falter, and the coordinated agency efforts, innovative research, and family-professional partnerships that have been created in the past decade could break down. Dismantling these efforts and starting over is highly inefficient and impractical. Instead, the most efficient, logical, and hopeful course is to maintain and strengthen what has already been set in place, is working well, and simply needs to be expanded and made sustainable. It is not only possible, but ethically imperative, that efforts continue to significantly improve outcomes for individuals with FASDs. These efforts can reduce the drain on emotional, physical, and financial resources that have devastated too many families and strained service delivery systems.

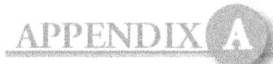

Action Steps for Recommendations of the National Task Force on Fetal Alcohol Syndrome and Fetal Alcohol Effect

1. **Modify eligibility and diagnostic classification systems to include FASDs, so as to recognize FASDs as approved conditions under all federal disability-related benefit programs.**

   - Modify Medicaid and insurance coding policies to appropriately fund screening, diagnosis, treatment, and support services for individuals with FASDs.
   - Make the following changes to the Child Abuse & Prevention Act (CAPTA) provision:
     — Add "and prenatal alcohol exposure" to the current CAPTA provision that requires referral to early intervention by social services and healthcare providers of children born drug-exposed.
     — Expand the age of referral to Child Find and early intervention services for children to "up to age five" in the current CAPTA provision.
   - Amend the recently reauthorized Individuals with Disabilities Education Act (IDEA) of 2004:
     — Include individuals with FASDs for eligibility under Part C and Part B.
     — Include technical assistance related to identifying children and youth with FASDs in Part D.
   - Work toward consensus on objective diagnostic criteria for the full fetal alcohol spectrum.
   - Directly and fully respond to FASDs in the classification systems of the widely-used psychiatric Diagnostic and Statistical Manual of Mental Disorders (American Psychiatric Association, 1994; now under revision), and the medical International Code for Diseases (ICD-10) (World Health Organization, 2005).

2. **Improve diagnostic access by setting up screening systems for FASDs and increasing professional multidisciplinary diagnostic capacity in communities.**

   - Require that critical systems with points of entry and exit set up effective strategies for screening, referral and treatment planning.[1]
   - Ensure local access to screening by requiring training on awareness of FASDs for providers in systems where screening takes place.
   - Promote regional access to appropriate multidisciplinary diagnostic and treatment services that reduce drive-time and waiting lists for families, including (when feasible and efficient) specialized FASD diagnostic clinics.
   - Ensure that efforts toward FASD prevention, substance use education, and referral for chemical dependency treatment are included in FASD diagnostic services.

3. **Intensify research initiatives and interagency coordination to:**

   - Delineate the full fetal alcohol spectrum, including fetal alcohol syndrome (FAS), partial FAS, and alcohol-related neurodevelopmental disorder (ARND).
   - Work toward consensus on objective diagnostic criteria for the full fetal alcohol spectrum.
   - Continue study of alcohol mechanisms and the impact of intervention using animal models.
   - Improve understanding of the mechanisms of alcohol's action on the brain through neuroimaging and basic science studies.
   - Enhance prevention and early detection through research to identify maternal and fetal biomarkers.
   - Improve understanding of neuroprotective factors.
   - Study the long-term, natural developmental course of individuals with FASDs.
   - Identify and test useful instructional methods for individuals with FASDs.
   - Create and establish the efficacy of intervention approaches for individuals with FASDs and their caregivers (including behavioral, psychopharmacology, and combined treatments).
   - Translate effective identification, diagnosis, and intervention strategies to community settings.
   - Improve the quality and utilization of interventions in all services systems for those with FASDs.

4. **Promote a comprehensive and accessible continuum of care for families raising infants, children and adolescents with FASDs.**

   - Require updated education and training for healthcare, mental health providers, early interventionists, and educators on: FASDs; the family perspective; identification, referral and effective intervention; and how to emphasize functional life skills.
   - Promote caregiver stress reduction through increased access to flexible respite care services.
   - Establish a continuum of scientifically tested or promising interventions, specialized for FASDs, that can address the full range of severity of family needs and child/adolescent problems:

---

[1]Critical systems with points of entry and exit that need to set up effective strategies for screening, referral and treatment planning: newborn screening, early periodic screening, diagnosis and treatment (EPSDT), early intervention, child welfare and foster care, special education, family court proceedings, juvenile and criminal justice, WIC programs, inpatient psychiatric care, and chemical dependency treatment.

— For example: Parent-to-parent support, parenting groups, child groups, social skills training, teen groups and retreats, summer camps, ongoing individualized behavioral and/or learning readiness consultation services for families with children at high risk, parent-child assistance programs for women with chemical dependency problems, direct child treatments (e.g., computer training, self-regulation techniques), special instructional programming and school behavior plans.

5. **Promote a comprehensive and accessible continuum of care for youth, adults and older individuals with FASDs.**

   • Modify eligibility for existing vocational and supported living/housing services to include individuals with FASDs (which may include altering current IQ and functional level requirements).

   • Promote creation of strength-based programs that include protective oversight as well as gradual, supported progressive skill-building (e.g., mentoring programs, supported living).

   • Develop and use appropriate alternative strategies within juvenile justice systems and corrections programs to ensure safety and effective diversion or rehabilitation of individuals with FASDs.

   • Recognize that FASDs can be a "transgenerational" problem—with affected individuals becoming involved in substance use and sexual activity, and so at risk for (or having) affected children. Because of this, promote specialized, intensive FASD prevention, chemical dependency treatment, and parenting support programs for youth and adults with FASDs.

6. **Encourage comprehensive professional education on FASDs, and assessment of knowledge gained, within multiple service systems.**[2]

   • Provide technical assistance on FASDs through specialized regional training centers and federal technical assistance systems.

   • Include information on FASDs in pre-service training, board examinations, licensing mechanisms, and continuing education for providers in multiple service systems.

7. **Enhance strong, collaborative, interagency leadership at state and national levels (that includes parent representation) to inform legislators, policymakers, and the public.**

   • Maintain high-level interagency coordination activities, such as those of the Interagency Coordinating Committee for FAS (ICCFAS).

   • Promote coordinated state systems to respond to FASDs, including appointing state-level FASD coordinators following the lead of SAMHSA initiatives.

   • Establish or maintain a lead federal agency to promote field-initiated and translational research and facilitate comprehensive systems of care over the lifespan.

8. **Recognize grassroots family support and advocacy organizations focused on FASDs, which are powerful and efficient agents of change.**

   • Use existing FASD organizations to educate and monitor policy. Possible actions: host U.S. House and Senate briefings; sponsor FASD Education Days; conduct personal meetings with legislators.

   • Disseminate state-of-the-art research and policy changes through existing databases and websites.

   • Maintain the FASD Caucus in the U.S. Senate, promoting and monitoring membership.

   • Maintain the organized birth mother/family movement to promote FASD prevention and support for recovery from addiction.

   • Maintain an organized effort to continue communication to family groups and coalitions about gains from FASD prevention, diagnosis and treatment, and remaining prevention, diagnostic, and treatment needs.

9. **Improve ongoing national surveillance systems to identify individuals with FASDs to better track prevalence, provide needed intervention, and assess the impact of prevention programs.**

   • Increase the number of states carrying out surveillance of FAS and partial FAS, especially: effective, active surveillance, and incorporating FAS/PFAS into existing birth defects surveillance systems.

   • When identification methods become available, increase the number of states carrying out effective, active surveillance of alcohol-related neurodevelopmental disorder (ARND).

10. **Maintain a national forum in which parents, advocates, professional organizations, and experts in the field of FASDs can work to advance essential services and research for individuals with FASDs and their families.**

---

[2] Target service systems in need of comprehensive professional education on FASDs, and assessment of knowledge gained: health care (obstetrics/gynecology, pediatrics, internal medicine, family practice, nursing), allied professions (occupational therapy, speech-language pathology), mental health (e.g., psychiatry, psychology, social work, counseling), early intervention, regular and special education, child welfare, developmental disabilities, vocational services, juvenile justice and corrections, and chemical dependency treatment.

Accomplishments of the National Task Force on Fetal Alcohol Syndrome and Fetal Alcohol Effect

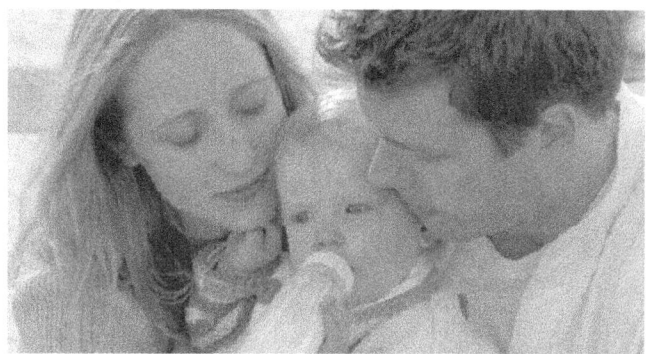

BACKGROUND

In 1998, the U.S. Congress recognized the significance of a coordinated effort to address the concerns related to FAS and fetal alcohol effects (FAE). The Secretary of the U.S. Department of Health and Human Services (DHHS) was directed through the Public Health Service Act, Section 399G (42 U.S.C. Section 280f, as added by Public Law 105-392) to establish a National Task Force on Fetal Alcohol Syndrome and Fetal Alcohol Effect (the Task Force) that would: (1) foster coordination among all governmental agencies, academic bodies, and community groups that conduct or support FAS and FAE research, programs, and surveillance; and (2) otherwise meet the needs of populations impacted by FAS and FAE. On May 17, 2000, in accordance with Public Law 92-463, the Task Force was chartered. Authority to establish the Task Force was delegated to CDC's National Center on Birth Defects and Developmental Disabilities (NCBDDD). NCBDDD's Fetal Alcohol Syndrome Prevention Team was assigned primary responsibility for establishing the Task Force and managing its operations. The Task Force function, as outlined in its charter (DHHS, 2000), is to:

- Advise persons involved in federal, state, and local programs and research activities of FAS and FAE regarding such topics as FAS awareness and education for relevant service providers and the general public (including school-aged children and women at risk), medical diagnosis for FAS and FAE, prevention and intervention strategies for women at risk, and essential services for affected persons and their families;
- Coordinate its efforts with the DHHS Interagency Coordinating Committee on Fetal Alcohol Syndrome (ICCFAS); and
- Report, on a biennial basis, to the DHHS Secretary and relevant committees of Congress on the current and planned activities of the participating agencies.

SELECTED ACCOMPLISHMENTS

- The Task Force outlined a national agenda for FAS and other prenatal alcohol-related conditions in a 2002 MMWR Recommendations and Reports publication, *National Task Force on Fetal Alcohol Syndrome and Fetal Alcohol Effect: Defining a National Agenda for Fetal Alcohol Syndrome and Other Prenatal Alcohol Related Disorders (MMWR, 2002).*
- Several Task Force members participated on the Scientific Working Group (SWG) on Diagnostic Guidelines for FAS and ARND Meeting in July 2002, provided input in various SWG committees, and deliberated on and approved *Fetal Alcohol Syndrome: Guidelines on Referral and Diagnosis (Bertrand, et al., 2004).*
- Recommendations were sent to the Office of Education to include FAS in the reauthorization of the Individuals with Disabilities in Education Act (IDEA) of 2004.
- In 2004, the Task Force endorsed the consensus definition of the term "fetal alcohol spectrum disorders" (FASDs) developed through an expert panel convened by the National Organization on Fetal Alcohol Syndrome.
- In 2005, the Task Force supported efforts to bring FASDs to the attention of the American Psychiatric Association in its deliberations on the 5th Edition of the *Diagnostic and Statistical Manual of Mental Disorders.*
- Task Force recommended an updated release of the Surgeon General's advisory on alcohol and pregnancy in 2001. This request was reviewed and approved by the Task Force and received key federal agency support. The Surgeon General's *Advisory on Alcohol Use in Pregnancy* was released in 2005 (Office of the Surgeon General, 2005). Task Force and liaison members, along with various federal agencies, were also involved in activities to disseminate the Advisory.
- *A Call to Action: Advancing Essential Services and Research on Fetal Alcohol Spectrum Disorders* was developed and approved by the Task Force in 2007. This document emphasizes the importance of early identification, diagnostic services, and quality research on interventions for individuals with FASDs and their families. Recommendations on continuing and enhancing these kinds of activities are outlined.

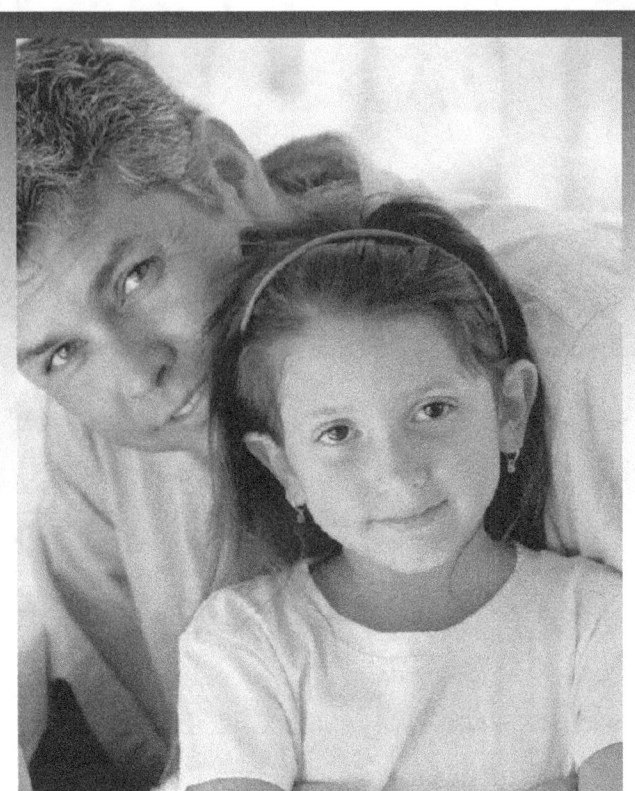

- *Reducing Alcohol-Exposed Pregnancies: A Report of the National Task Force on Fetal Alcohol Syndrome and Fetal Alcohol Effect* was developed and approved by the Task Force in 2007. This report reviews current evidence on prevention strategies to reduce alcohol use and alcohol-exposed pregnancies, provides recommendations on promoting and improving these strategies, and offers future research directions in the field of FASD prevention.

For more information, see National Task Force on Fetal Alcohol Syndrome and Fetal Alcohol Effect web site. http://www.cdc.gov/ncbddd/fas/taskforce.htm

REFERENCES

Bertrand J, Floyd RL, Weber MK, O'Connor M, Riley EP, Johnson KA, Cohen DE, NTFFAS/E. (2004). Fetal Alcohol Syndrome: Guidelines for Referral and Diagnosis. Atlanta, GA: Centers for Disease Control and Prevention.

Centers for Disease Control and Prevention. National Task Force on Fetal Alcohol Syndrome and Fetal Alcohol Effect --- Defining the national agenda for fetal alcohol syndrome and other prenatal alcohol-related effects (2002). MMWR Morbidity and Mortality Weekly Report Recommendations and Report: 51(RR14):9-12.

Department of Health & Human Services. (2000). Charter: National Task Force on Fetal Alcohol Syndrome and Fetal Alcohol Effect. Rockville, MD: US DHHS, Office of the Secretary,p. 1-3. http://www.cdc.gov/ncbddd/fas/charter.htm.

Office of the Surgeon General. (2005). Surgeon General's Advisory on Alcohol Use in Pregnancy. http://www.cdc.gov/ncbddd/fas/documents/Released%20Advisory.pdf

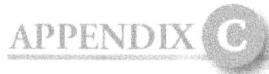
Overview of the Strategic Research Plan on FASDs from the National Institute on Alcohol Abuse and Alcoholism

OVERVIEW

The National Institute on Alcohol Abuse and Alcoholism (NIAAA) is one of the 27 Institutes and Centers which comprise the National Institutes of Health, "The Nation's Medical Research Agency," a component of the U. S. Department of Health and Human Services. The NIAAA is the primary U.S. agency for conducting and supporting research on the causes, consequences, prevention, and treatment of alcohol abuse, alcoholism, and alcohol problems— and the NIAAA disseminates research findings to general, professional, and academic audiences.

The NIAAA mission is to provide leadership in the national effort to reduce alcohol-related problems by:

- Conducting and supporting research in a wide range of scientific areas including genetics, neuroscience, epidemiology, health risks and benefits of alcohol consumption, prevention, and treatment
- Coordinating and collaborating with other research institutes and Federal Programs on alcohol-related issues
- Collaborating with international, national, state, and local institutions, organizations, agencies, and programs engaged in alcohol-related work
- Translating and disseminating research findings to health care providers, researchers, policymakers, and the public

The NIAAA's efforts to fulfill its mission are guided by the Director's Vision to support and promote the best science on alcohol and health for the benefit of all by:

- Increasing the understanding of normal and abnormal biological functions and behavior relating to alcohol use
- Improving the diagnosis, prevention, and treatment of alcohol use disorders
- Enhancing quality health care

Since the initial U.S. discovery of the detrimental effects of prenatal alcohol exposure, a substantial portion of the NIAAA research budget has been dedicated each year to research on FASD-related issues. The NIAAA research portfolio includes projects whose goals are prevention of drinking during pregnancy, increased understanding of the etiology of alcohol-attributable fetal injury, better diagnosis of FASD, and development of interventions to reduce the effects of prenatal alcohol exposure, mitigate the consequences of alcohol-induced injury, and improve the quality of life for persons with FASD. Furthermore, the NIAAA research portfolio on prevention of alcohol use disorders supports prevention research studies specifically aimed at reduction of drinking by both non-pregnant and pregnant women of childbearing age. The NIAAA supports the activities of the Interagency Coordinating Committee on Fetal Alcohol Syndrome (ICCFAS) and collaborates with many other federal agencies whose missions and/or program interests include FASD. In addition to conducting and supporting FASD-related research the NIAAA also regularly produces publications summarizing research results, clinical guidelines, and educational materials relevant to FASD. Check the NIAAA Web site for the most recent version of the NIAAA Strategic Plan, more details about the FASD research program, and currently available publications: http://www.niaaa.nih.gov/

For more information, see:
National Institute on Alcohol Abuse and Alcoholism (NIAAA). (2006, July).
NIAAA: Five-year strategic plan (FY 07-11): Alcohol across the lifespan. http://pubs.niaaa.nih.gov/publications/StrategicPlan/NIAAASTRATEGICPLAN.htm

See also the link to research aims specifically for study of FAS and prenatal alcohol exposure, as it applies to health disparities:
http://www.niaaa.nih.gov/AboutNIAAA/OrganizationalInformation/HealthDisparities2005.htm

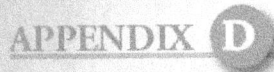

Activities of the Centers for Disease Control and Prevention Related to Fetal Alcohol Spectrum Disorders

Fetal Alcohol Syndrome Prevention Team
Prevention Research Branch
Division of Birth Defects and Developmental Disabilities
National Center on Birth Defects and
Developmental Disabilities

MISSION

The mission of the Centers for Disease Control and Prevention's (CDC) Fetal Alcohol Syndrome (FAS) Prevention Team is to prevent FAS and other prenatal alcohol-related conditions and ameliorate these conditions in children already affected.

BACKGROUND/OVERVIEW

CDC has been involved in FAS-related activities since 1991. The FAS Prevention Team resides in the National Center on Birth Defects and Developmental Disabilities, Division of Birth Defects and Developmental Disabilities, at CDC. Recently, the FAS Prevention Team became part of the Prevention Research Branch, one of three branches within the division. The FAS Prevention Team currently funds a total of 26 cooperative agreements in 18 states, as well as 3 international projects. Some of these cooperative agreements also reach out to additional states.

FAS PREVENTION TEAM EFFORTS

The FAS Prevention Team works to develop systems to monitor exposures and outcomes; to conduct epidemiologic studies and public health research to identify maternal risk factors associated with giving birth to a child with FAS or another prenatal alcohol-related condition, known collectively as fetal alcohol spectrum disorders (FASDs); and to implement and evaluate prevention and intervention programs.

Current activities include:
- Prevention efforts
  - Implementing state-based FASD prevention projects
  - Conducting intervention research for preventing alcohol-exposed pregnancies
  - Identifying alcohol-exposed pregnancies through biomarkers
- Monitoring efforts
  - Tracking alcohol use among childbearing-aged women
  - Establishing and guiding the implementation of surveillance systems for the prevalence of FAS through state-based projects
  - Assessing health care providers' knowledge, attitudes, and practices regarding screening for alcohol use, provision of brief interventions, and care of individuals with FASDs
- Interventions for children with FASDs
  - Implementing tested intervention strategies for children living with FASDs in community-based settings
- Education efforts
  - Supporting FASD Regional Training Centers for medical and allied health students and practitioners
  - Developing screening and intervention tools for women's health care providers
  - Responding to public inquiries and disseminate educational materials to various audiences
- International efforts in South Africa, Denmark, and Russia
- Partner engagement
  - Coordinating the National Task Force on Fetal Alcohol Syndrome and Fetal Alcohol Effect
  - Promoting various collaborations with internal and external partners

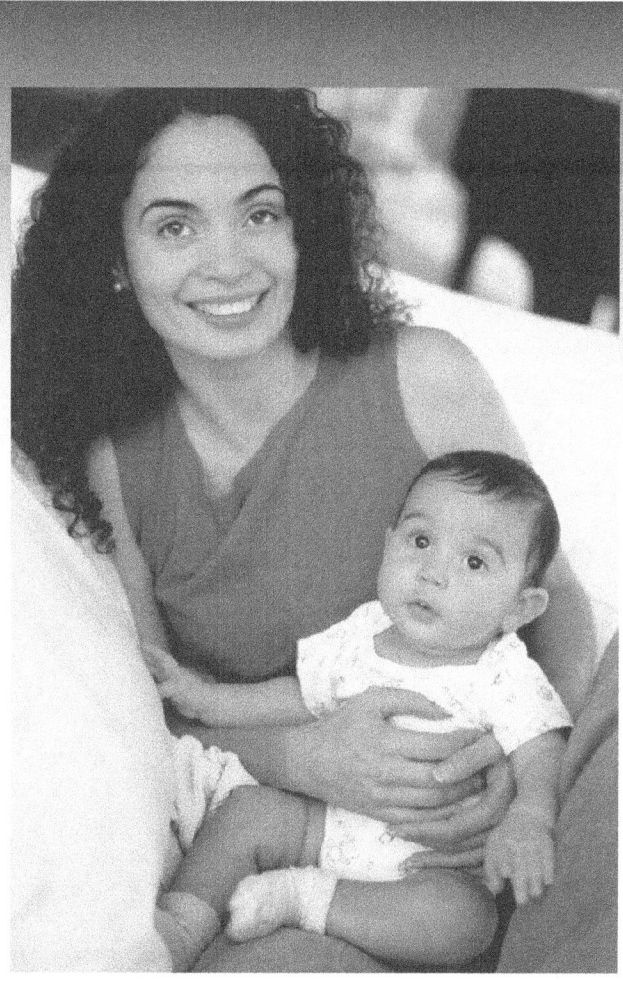

Recent Accomplishments

- Developing *Fetal Alcohol Syndrome: Guidelines for Referral and Diagnosis* in 2004.
- Participation in implementing the 2005 U.S. Surgeon General's *Advisory on Alcohol Use in Pregnancy*, in collaboration with the National Task Force on Fetal Alcohol Syndrome and Fetal Alcohol Effect, relevant federal agencies, and other partners.
- Developing and disseminating of a tool kit for women's health care providers, in partnership with the American College of Obstetricians and Gynecologists, in 2006. This tool kit helps providers screen female patients for risky drinking and deliver brief interventions for those at risk for an alcohol-exposed pregnancy.
- Completing Project CHOICES (2007), which found that women who received brief motivational counseling sessions were twice as likely to reduce their risk for an alcohol-exposed pregnancy as women who did not receive the counseling. Risk was reduced either by decreasing alcohol use, by using more effective contraception, or both.
- Developing systematic, specific, and scientifically evaluated interventions for children with FASDs currently underway.

Future Directions

- Exploring the feasibility of establishing ongoing FAS surveillance as part of the National Birth Defects Prevention Network and the Metropolitan Atlanta Congenital Defects Program.
- Promoting continued dialogue with the FASD field regarding diagnostic criteria for prenatal alcohol-related conditions other than FAS.
- Continuing to monitor alcohol consumption rates among women of childbearing age.
- Conducting epidemiological studies to identify other risk factors commonly found in combination with the risk for an alcohol-exposed pregnancy.
- Exploring the effect of multiple-risk factor interventions on reducing alcohol-exposed pregnancies.
- Conducting further testing of the Project Choices intervention model targeting women in diverse, population-based settings not previously studied (e.g., American Indian/Alaska Native populations, worksite programs, health insurance agencies)
- Packaging and disseminating the Project CHOICES intervention for various public health and social service audiences.
- Expanding the translation of CDC's model programs for intervening with children with FASDs and their families.
- Continuing to support provider education regarding the recognition of FASDs and the identification of women at risk for an alcohol-exposed pregnancy.
- Continuing to inform consumers, health providers, and other groups about FASDs and the risks of drinking alcohol during pregnancy.

To learn more about FASDs and CDC's FASD program activities, visit http://www.cdc.gov/ncbddd/fas/ or http://www.cdc.gov/ncbddd/fas/cdcactivities.htm.

Overview of the Substance Abuse and Mental Health Services Administration's FASD Center for Excellence

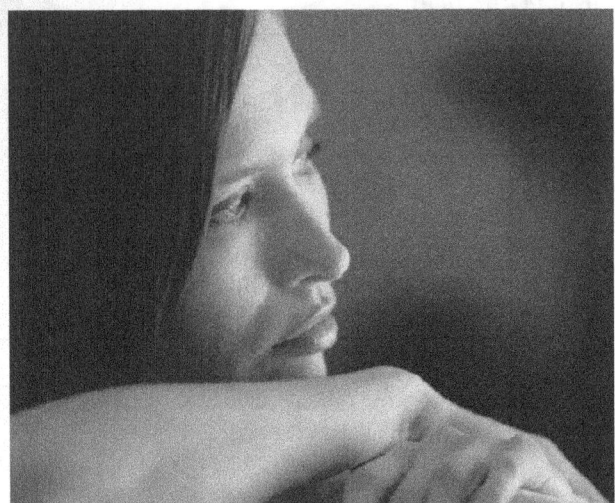

The Substance Abuse and Mental Health Services Administration (SAMHSA), United States Department of Health and Human Services (HHS), is the lead Federal agency addressing substance abuse and mental health services. SAMHSA's mission is to build resilience and facilitate recovery for people with or at risk for substance abuse and mental illness. SAMHSA was established as a services agency in 1992, though its predecessors have existed within the Public Health Service since 1930.

The SAMHSA FASD Center for Excellence was launched in 2001. Congress authorized the Center in Section 519D of the Children's Health Act of 2000, which included six mandates (Section b of 42 USC 290bb-25d or Public Law 106-310). The mandates focus on exploring innovative service delivery strategies, developing comprehensive systems of care for FASD prevention and treatment, training service system staff, families, and individuals with an FASD, and preventing alcohol use among women of childbearing age.

MISSION STATEMENT

The mission of the FASD Center for Excellence is to facilitate the development and improvement of prevention, treatment, and care systems in the United States by providing national leadership and facilitating collaboration in the field.

Vision of the FASD Center

1. Reduce the number of infants born prenatally exposed to alcohol.
2. Increase functioning of persons who have an FASD.
3. Improve quality of life for individuals and families affected by FASD.

Goals of the FASD Center

1. Facilitate the development of FASD prevention, treatment, and care as a specialty field.
2. Facilitate the development of FASD prevention, treatment, and care systems at the State and community level.

For more information, see: http://www.fasdcenter.samhsa.gov/

Information about the Interagency Coordinating Committee on Fetal Alcohol Syndrome

The Interagency Coordinating Committee on Fetal Alcohol Syndrome (ICCFAS) was created in October of 1996, in response to a report by an expert committee of the Institute of Medicine (IOM). The IOM report is entitled *Fetal Alcohol Syndrome: Diagnosis, Epidemiology, Prevention, and Treatment (Stratton et al., 1996)*. The report recommended that the National Institute on Alcohol Abuse and Alcoholism (NIAAA) chair a federal effort to coordinate fetal alcohol syndrome (FAS) activities, because the responsibility for addressing the many issues relevant to FAS transcends the mission and resources of any single agency or program. The ICCFAS is chaired by a member of the Senior Staff of the NIAAA.

The mission of the ICCFAS is to enhance and increase communication, cooperation, collaboration, and partnerships among disciplines and federal agencies to address health, education, developmental disabilities, alcohol research, and health and social services and justice issues that are relevant to disorders caused by prenatal alcohol exposure. The themes around which the ICCFAS bases the foundation of its current work are: (1) prevention of drinking during pregnancy; (2) intervening with children and families affected by prenatal alcohol exposure; (3) improving methods for diagnosis and case identification; (4) increasing research on etiology and pathogenesis; and (5) increasing information dissemination. The vision of ICCFAS is that collaborative partnerships, using the resources of governmental and other organizations, will reduce the prevalence of individuals affected by prenatal exposure to alcohol, provide appropriate interventions and support to persons affected by fetal alcohol spectrum disorders (FASD) and their families, and build sustainable approaches within existing systems to properly address the disorders.

Communication, collaboration, and cooperation are fostered and promoted among ICCFAS members through meetings, informal discussions, and the overall exchange of ideas and updates of new findings and activities in conversations and electronic missives. Strategies on how activities in different agencies can complement each other and how synergy can be achieved are the primary focus of these exchanges. Leveraging the work of member organizations through more collaborative and cooperative activities is a key strategy. The concept of distributed leadership is used to increase cooperation and collaboration within the ICCFAS agencies on projects of mutual interest.

The ICCFAS increases communication among participating organizations via shared meetings, workshops, planning sessions, and formal information exchanging sessions. Collaboration has been increased by co-sponsorship of conferences, research programs, observational studies, and outreach activities. Cooperation has been increased by representatives from ICCFAS member agencies providing service to each other as speakers at conferences, meetings, and workshops and in writing articles for newsletters sponsored by other participating organizations. Furthermore, ICCFAS members provide assistance as advisors and consultants to fellow members and their agencies. These advisory and consultant roles have been in the form of service on formal advisory committees, help with preparation of program announcements and requests for applications, review of proposals, and assistance in launching outreach programs. The membership of the ICCAFS is dynamic, changing as federal agencies emphasize different aspects of their missions. The FY2007 membership of the ICCFAS included representatives from the following organizations:

- Department of Justice (DOJ), Office of Juvenile Justice and Delinquency Prevention (OJJDP)
- Department of Education (ED), Office of Special Education and Rehabilitative Services (OSERS)
- Department of Health and Human Services (DHHS)
  — Agency for Heathcare Research and Quality (AHRQ)
  — Centers for Disease Control and Prevention (CDC)
  — Health Resources and Services Administration (HRSA)
  — Indian Health Service (IHS)
  — Substance Abuse and Mental Health Services Administration (SAMHSA)
  — National Institutes of Health (NIH):
    – National Institute on Alcohol Abuse and Alcoholism (NIAAA)
    – National Institute of Child Health and Human Development (NICHD)

The member organizations have diverse missions and unique strengths. Some generate new knowledge through research funding. Other agencies fund translational research that feeds back to promote basic research. Others promote and assist in the development and improvement of health care delivery services by states and community organizations. One of the guiding principles of the ICCFAS has been to use the diverse missions, strengths, and resources of the various member organizations to advance the effectiveness of the federal response to alcohol-related birth defects. The ICCFAS implements its policy of shared leadership through use of subcommittees and working groups led by different agencies to help set direction and apprise the ICCFAS of new opportunities for action in specific areas.

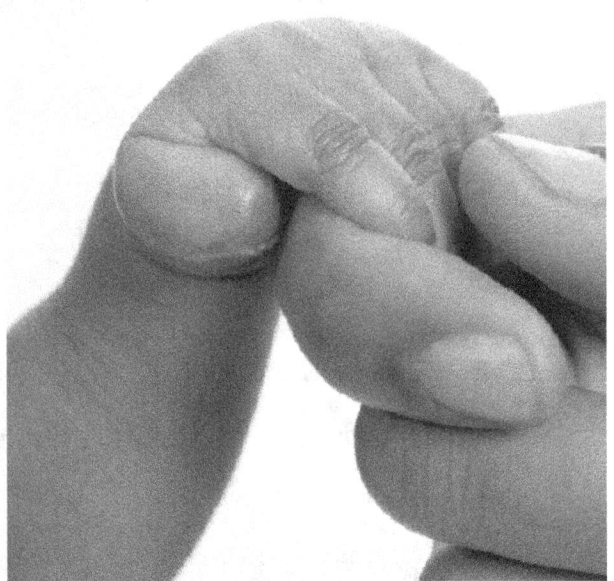

The ICCFAS Work Groups (subcommittees) address special issues and implementation of planned activities. Work Groups allow the membership of the ICCFAS to work with a lead agency and some outside experts to plan and develop actions on a specific issue. The Work Groups are usually composed of several members of the ICCFAS and/other representatives from member federal agencies, and six or seven individuals who are knowledgeable about FASD but are not part of the U.S. government. A broad perspective and balance on the ICCFAS Work Groups is assured by including biomedical researchers, physicians and other service providers, educators, FASD advocates, and other interested and knowledgeable persons. In FY2007 there were three ICCFAS Work Groups: ICCFAS Work Group on Women, Drinking, and Pregnancy; ICCFAS Work Group on Juvenile Justice Issues; and the ICCFAS Education Work Group.

Check the ICCFAS web page at the NIAAA website for information on current membership, links to members' websites, current activities, meeting summaries, resource materials, proceedings of conferences, and progress reports.

For more information, see:
http://www.niaaa.nih.gov/AboutNIAAA/InterAgency/

REFERENCES

Adnams, C.M., Sorour, P., Kalberg, W.O., Kodituwakku, P., Perold, M.D., et al. (2007). Language and literacy outcomes from a pilot intervention study for children with fetal alcohol spectrum disorders in South Africa. Alcohol, 41(6), 403-414.

Alcohol Research & Health. (2000). Highlights from the 10th Special Report to Congress. Chapter on Prenatal exposure to alcohol. Alcohol Research & Health, 24(1), 32-41.

American Academy of Pediatrics. (2000). Committee on Substance Abuse and Committee on Children with Disabilities. Fetal alcohol syndrome and alcohol-related neurodevelopmental disorders. Pediatrics, 106, 358-361.

American College of Obstetricians & Gynecologists (ACOG). (2005). Substance use: Obstetric and gynecologic implications. ACOG Special Issues in Women's Health, 105-150. ACOG: Washington DC.

American College of Obstetricians & Gynecologists (ACOG). (2006). Drinking and reproductive health: A fetal alcohol spectrum disorders toolkit (with CD-ROM). Washington, D.C.: American College of Obstetricians & Gynecologists. Also published on the ACOG website: http://www.acog.org/from_home/misc/dept_pubs.cfm. Accessed 2/26/07.

American Psychiatric Association. (1994). Diagnostic and statistical manual of mental disorders. (4th ed). Washington, DC: American Psychiatric Association.

Barry K.L., Caetano R., Chang G., DeJoseph M.C., Miller L.A., O'Connor M.J., Olson H.C., Floyd R.L., Weber M.K., DeStefano F., Dolina S., Leeks K., National Task Force on Fetal Alcohol Syndrome and Fetal Alcohol Effect. Reducing alcohol-exposed pregnancies: A report of the National Task Force on Fetal Alcohol Syndrome and Fetal Alcohol Effect. Atlanta, GA: Centers for Disease Control and Prevention, March 2009.

Bertrand, J., Floyd, R.L., Weber, M.K., O'Connor. M., Riley, E.P., Johnson, K.A., & Cohen, D.E. (2004). Fetal Alcohol Syndrome: Guidelines for Referral and Diagnosis. Atlanta, GA: Centers for Disease Control and Prevention.

Bonthius, D.J., Olson, H.C. & Thomas. J. (2006). Proceedings of the 2006 annual meeting of the Fetal Alcohol Spectrum Disorders Study Group. Alcohol, 40(1), 61-65.

Burden, M.J., Jacobson, S.W. & Jacobson. J.L. (2005). Relationship of prenatal alcohol exposure to cognitive processing speed and efficiency in childhood. Alcoholism: Clinical & Experimental Research, 29(8), 1473-1483.

Calhoun, F., Attilia, M.L., Spagnolo, P.A., Rotondo, C., Mancinelli, R. & Ceccanti, M. (2006). National Institute on Alcohol Abuse and Alcoholism and the study of fetal alcohol spectrum disorders. The International Consortium. Annali dell'Instituto Superiore di Sanita, 42(1), 4-7.

Centers for Disease Control and Prevention. (2004). Alcohol consumption among women who are pregnant or might become pregnant—United States, 2002. MMRW Morbidity & Mortality Weekly Report, 53(50), 1178-1181.

Chang, G., McNamara, Orav, E.J. (2005). Brief intervention for prenatal alcohol use: A randomized trial. Obstetrics & Gynecology, 105, 991-998.

Chudley, A.E., Conry, J., Cook, J.L., Loock, C., Rsales, T., & LeBlanc, N. Public Health Agency of Canada's National Advisory Committee on Fetal Alcohol Spectrum Disorder. (2005). Fetal alcohol spectrum disorder: Canadian guidelines for diagnosis. Canadian Medicine Journal, 172(5 Suppl), S1-S21.

Coles, C.D., Strickland, D.C., Padgett, L. & Bellmoff, L. (2006). Games that "work:" Using computer games to teach alcohol-affected children about fire and street safety. Research in Developmental Disabilities, advance online publication, 9 Sep 2006; doi:10.1016/j.ridd/2006.07.001

Coles, C.D., Kable, J.A., Taddeo, E. (2009). Math performance and behavior problems in children affected by prenatal alcohol exposure: Intervention and follow-up. Journal of Developmental & Behavioral Pediatrics, 30, 7-15.

Finer, L. B., & Henshaw, S. K. (2006). Disparities in rates of unintended pregnancy in the United States, 1994 and 2001. Perspectives on Sexual and Reproductive Health, 38(2), 90-96.

Floyd, R.L., O'Connor, M.J., Bertrand, J. & Sokol, R. (2006). Reducing adverse outcomes from prenatal alcohol exposure: A clinical plan of action. Alcoholism: Clinical & Experimental Research, 30(8), 1271-1275.

Floyd R.L., Sobell M., Velasquez M., Ingersoll K., et al. (2007). Preventing alcohol-exposed pregnancies: a randomized controlled trial. American Journal of Preventive Medicine, 32(1), 1-10.

Gemma, S., Vichi, S & Testai, E. (2007). Metabolic and genetic factors contributing to alcohol induced effects and fetal alcohol syndrome. Neuroscience & Biobehavioral Reviews, 31, 221-229.

Grant, T.M, Ernst C.C., Streissguth, A. & Stark, K. (2005). Preventing alcohol and drug exposed births in Washington state: Intervention findings from three parent-child assistance program sites. The American Journal of Drug & Alcohol Abuse, 31(3), 471-490.

Hankin, J.R. (2002). Fetal alcohol syndrome prevention research. Alcohol Research & Health, 26(1), 58-65.

Hannigan, J.H., O'Leary-Moore, S.K, Berman, R.F. (2007). Postnatal environmental or experiential amelioration of neurobehavioral effects of perinatal alcohol exposure in rats, Neuroscience & Biobehavioral Reviews, 31, 202-211.

Individuals with Disabilities Education Act (IDEA). Individuals with Disabilities Improvement Act of 2004, 20 U.S.C.A § 1400 et seq. (Thomson-West, 2005). [PL 108-46].

Interventions for Children with Fetal Alcohol Spectrum Disorders Research Consortium. (in press). Interventions for children with fetal alcohol spectrum disorders: Overview of findings for five innovative research projects. Research in Developmental Disabilities.

Jacobson, J.L. & Jacobson, S.W. (1999). Drinking moderately and pregnancy: Effects on child development. Alcohol Health & Research World, 23, 25-30.

Kable, J.A., Coles, C.D. & Taddeo, E. (2007). Sociocognitive habilitation using the math interactive learning experience program for alcohol-affected children. Alcoholism: Clinical & Experimental Research, 31(8), 1425-1434.

Kalberg, W.O. & Buckley, D. (2007). FASD: What types of intervention and rehabilitation are useful? Neuroscience & Biobehavioral Reviews, 31, 278-285.

Keeping Children and Families Safe Act of 2003, 42 U.S.C.A § 670 et seq. (Thomson-West, 2003). [Child Abuse Prevention and Treatment Act (CAPTA) PL. 93-247 as amended by Keeping Children and Families Safe Act of 2003 Pl 108-36.]

Kodituwakku, P.W. (2007). Defining the behavioral phenotype in children with fetal alcohol spectrum disorders. Neuroscience & Biobehavioral Reviews, 31, 192-201.

Lupton, C., Burd, L. & Harwood, R. (2004). Cost of fetal alcohol spectrum disorders. American Journal of Medical Genetics. Part C: Seminars in Medical Genetics, 127(1), 42-50.

Mattson, S. N., Riley, E. P., Gramling, L., Delis, D. C. & Jones, K. L. (1998). Neuropsychological comparison of alcohol exposed children with or without the physical features of fetal alcohol syndrome. Neuropsychology, 12(1), 16-153.

May, P.A., & Gossage, J.P. (2001). Estimating the prevalence of fetal alcohol syndrome: A summary. Alcohol Research & Health, 25, 159-167.

May, P.A., Fiorentino, D., Gossage, J.P., Kalberg, W.O., Hoyme, H.E., Robinson, L.K., et al. (2006). Epidemiology of FASD in a province in Italy: Prevalence and characteristics of children in a random sample of schools. Alcoholism and Clinical Experimental Research, 30(9), 1562-1575.

Miller, M.W. & Spear, L.P. (2006). The alcoholism generator. Alcoholism: Clinical & Experimental Research, 30(9), 1466-1469.

National Institute on Alcohol Abuse and Alcoholism (2005). Helping Patients who Drink Too Much: A Clinician's Guide. NIH Pub. No 05-3769.

O'Connor, M.J. & Whaley, S.E. (2007). Brief intervention for alcohol use by pregnant women. Am J Public Health, 97(2): p. 252-8.

O'Connor M.J., Frankel, F., Paley, B., Schonfeld, A.M., Carpenter, E., Laugeson, E., & Marquardt, R. (2006). A controlled social skills training for children with fetal alcohol spectrum disorders. Journal of Consulting & Clinical Psychology, 74, 639-48.

Office of the Surgeon General, U.S. Department of Health and Human Services. (2005). Advisory on alcohol use in pregnancy. Accessed June 16, 2007, from http://www.surgeongeneral.gov/pressreleases/sg02222005.html.

Olson, H. Carmichael. (2006). The current state of FASD intervention: An overview to spark debate and new ideas. Iceberg, 16 (4). Download from: http://fasiceberg.org/newsletters/Vol16Num4_Nov2006.htm#currentstate

Olson, H. Carmichael, Quamma, J., Brooks, A., Lehman, K., Ranna, M, & Astley, S. (2005). Efficacy of a new model of behavioral consultation for families raising school-aged children with FASD and behavior problems. Alcoholism: Clinical & Experimental Research, 28 (Suppl. 5), 718.

Olson, H.Carmichael, Jirikowic. T., Kartin. D., & Astley, S. (2007). Responding to the challenge of early intervention for fetal alcohol spectrum disorders. Infants & Young Children, 20(2), 172-189.

Paley, B., O'Connor, M.J., Frankel, F., & Marquardt, R. (2006). Predictors of stress in parents of children with fetal alcohol spectrum disorders. Journal of Developmental & Behavioral Pediatrics, 27(5), 396-404.

Riley, E.P., & McGee, C.L. (2005). Fetal Alcohol Spectrum Disorders: An overview with emphasis on changes in brain and behavior. Experimental Biology & Medicine, 230, 357-365

Ryan, D.M., Bonnett, D.M. & Gass, C.B. (2006). Sobering Thoughts: Town Hall Meetings on Fetal Alcohol Spectrum Disorders. American Journal of Public Health, 96(12), 2098-2101.

Sampson, P.D., Streissguth, A.P., Bookstein, F.L., Little, R.E., Clarren, S.K., Dehaene, P., Hanson, J.W. & Graham, J.M. Jr. (1997). Incidence of fetal alcohol syndrome and prevalence of alcohol-related neurodevelopmental disorder. Teratology, 56(5), 317-326.

Sokol, R.J., Janisse, J.J., Louis, J.M., Bailey, B.N., Ager, J., Jacobson, S.W. & Jacobson, J.L. (2007). Extreme prematurity: An alcohol-related birth effect. Alcoholism: Clinical & Experimental Research, 31(6), 1031-1037.

Spadoni, A.D., McGee, C.L., Fryer, S.L. & Riley, E.P. (2007). Neuroimaging and fetal alcohol spectrum disorders. Neuroscience & Biobehavioral Reviews, 31, 239-245.

Stratton, K., Howe, C., & Battaglia, F. (Eds.) (1996). Fetal alcohol syndrome: Diagnosis, epidemiology, prevention and treatment. Institute of Medicine. Washington DC: National Academy Press.

Streissguth, A. P., Bookstein, F. L., Barr, H. M., Sampson, P. D., O'Malley, K., & Young, J.K. (2004). Risk factors for adverse life outcomes for fetal alcohol syndrome and fetal alcohol effects. Journal of Developmental & Behavioral Pediatrics, 25(4), 228-238.

Streissguth, A.P. & O'Malley, K. (2000). Neuropsychiatric implications and long-term consequences of fetal alcohol spectrum disorders. Seminars in Clinic Neuropsychiatry, 5(3), 177-190.

Substance Abuse and Mental Health Services Administration. (2007). Results from the 2006 National Household Survey on Drug Abuse and Health: National Findings. Office of Applied Studies, NSDUH Series H-32, DHHS Publication No. SMA 07-4293. Rockville, MD.

U.S. Preventive Services Task Force. (2004). Screening and behavioral counseling interventions in primary care to reduce alcohol misuse: Recommendation statement. Annals of Internal Medicine, 140, 554-556.

Vaglenova, J., Pandiella, N., Wijayawardhane, N., Vaithlanathan, T., Birru, S., Breese, C., Supplramaniam, V. & Randal, C. (2007). Aniracetam reversed learning and memory deficits following prenatal ethanol exposure by modulating functions of synaptic AMPA receptors Neuropsychopharmacology, advance online publication, 4 July 2007; doi:10.1038/sj.npp.1301496.

Viljoen, D.L., Gossage, J.P., Brooke, L., Adnams, C.M., Jones, K.L., Robinson, L.K., Hoyme, E., et al. (2005). Fetal alcohol syndrome epidemiology in a South African community: A second study of a very high prevalence area. Journal of Studies on Alcohol and Drug Use, 66, 593-604.

Warren, K., Floyd, L., Calhoun, F., Stone, D., Bertrand, J., Streissguth, A. et al. (2004). Consensus statement on FASD. World Health Organization. (2005). ICD-10: International statistical classification of diseases and related health problems. (10th revision) (2nd ed). Geneva: World Health Organization.

Zhang, X., Sliwowska, J.H., & Weinberg, J. (2005). Prenatal alcohol exposure and fetal programming: Effects on neuroendocrine function and immune function. Experimental Biology & Medicine, 230(6), 376-388.

WEBSITES

Alaska Office of Fetal Alcohol Syndrome
http://www.hss.state.ak.us/fas/default.htm
Accessed 4/15/08.

Fetal Alcohol Spectrum Disorders Study Group (FASDSG)
FASDSG home page: http://rsoa.org/fas.html.
Accessed 4/15/08.

Fetal Alcohol Syndrome Regional Training Centers
Meharry Medical College (Nashville, TN); Morehouse School of Medicine (Atlanta, GA); University of Medicine and Dentistry of New Jersey (Newark, NJ); St. Louis University School of Medicine (St. Louis, MO); University of California at Los Angeles School of Medicine (Los Angeles, CA).
http://www.cdc.gov/ncbddd/fas/regional.htm
Accessed 4/15/08.

National Organization on Fetal Alcohol Syndrome (NOFAS)
Home page: http://www.nofas.org/default.aspx
Clearinghouse information: http://www.nofas.org/resource/default.aspx
Congressional caucus on FASDs: http://www.house.gov/pallone/fasd_caucus/welcome.shtml
Accessed 4/15/08.

SAMHSA's FASD Center for Excellence
http://fasdcenter.samhsa.gov
Accessed 4/15/08.

www.ingramcontent.com/pod-product-compliance
Lightning Source LLC
Chambersburg PA
CBHW081418170526
45166CB00010B/3398